Nourishing Space Within

Essentials of Self-Care

Allegra Hart, N.D.

Nourishing Space Within
Essentials of Self-Care
Allegra Hart, ND

Naturae Naturopathic Clinic PLLC
1417 Maiden Lane, Wenatchee WA 98801
www.naturaeclinic.com / info@naturaeclinic.com

Disclaimer
The purpose of this book is to educate and is not intended to replace individualized professional medical advice. Use of the information in this book is at the reader's discretion. Every effort has been made to ensure the accuracy of the information in this book. To obtain personalized medical advice about your individual health needs, please consult a qualified health care practitioner.

ISBN: 978-0-9962367-0-6

Printed in the U.S.A.

Gratitude

My amazing husband Brandon: you are my beacon light. Thank you for encouraging me to acknowledge and kindle my own light. Words cannot express my awe and gratitude for the honor of sharing my life with you.

My parents, Joseph and Merry: you built the foundation on which I grew, and you allowed me to find my voice. Your love and support are immeasurable. Mom, thank you for nourishing my love of learning and helping me share it with the world. Dad, thank you for helping me step back and assess ideas from all angles; this is how I found me.

Dickson Thom (ND, DDS): your teachings and guidance helped me open my doors and have the courage to walk through. You showed me that the medicine my soul longed for was powerful and deep.

Special Thanks: Kristy Allen, Lindsay Peternell and Daphne Gordon

Happiness is not something ready-made.

It comes from your own actions.

~Dalai Lama

Table of Contents

Introduction

Life in all its fullness is Mother
Nature obeyed.

~Dr. Weston A. Price

In this book, I hope to teach you that in learning to maintain your foundation of health, even in the busiest of times, you will learn to step back into balance with your natural rhythms. When you begin to make a few of the simple changes I have recommended, life will flow to meet you in the most amazing ways.

In today's world of perpetual motion, with everyone on the go, running from home to work to school and home again, meeting the needs of family, work and community, it can be difficult to find time to slow down. In your hurry, you may find no choice but to trade quality for convenience. As time passes, however, your health will pay the price. Stress, pain, and discomfort may begin to seem like a normal part of daily life.

We are taught to suppress and be violent with ourselves. It is imprinted on us at a very young age. The average toddler hears "no" dozens of times each day. We teach our children to suppress their emotions, ignore their pain and accept discomfort. But at what cost?

Emotion and pain are teachers of deep and powerful lessons. You need these lessons and they *will* be heard. When you ignore these messages, they get louder and more aggressive. This is typically when your life takes a turn for the worse. You may begin to feel like you are falling apart. By becoming aware of the cycle of hurting yourself for the sake of convenience or comfort, and by beginning to respect the natural ebb and flow of your rhythms and cycles, you can begin to harmonize with the world around you. You can begin to relax into life with ease.

Committing to building your health will make it easier to continue with a regular self-care routine even when life gets difficult and busy. Working on self-care will help you debunk the lie that you are unworthy, and it will teach you that you are definitely worth the time and effort it takes to get to know yourself. You will begin to thrive.

Let me tell you a little bit about my path. My personal journey has been long and winding. As a very young child, I experienced abuse. At that age, I did not have the tools to deal with it, let alone the ability to acknowledge the damage.

I did my very best to suppress my memories, as I consciously ignored the chaos building inside. By the time I was a teenager, I had been caught in a tailspin for years. I began to break down physically and mentally. I became disillusioned with my life and the world around me. Regular panic attacks seemed "normal" and my nervous system was keyed to be hyper-vigilant. I was incapacitated by intense physical pain that came and went without warning.

When I was 19, I began to investigate my disconnection with myself. I decided there must be more to life than the fear and anger that constantly ran through me. I saw sincerely happy people and knew nothing of their world. I knew there had to be more to life.

For the first time, I stepped back from my life and social interactions. I withdrew into solitude and silence when I was not at work. I turned to art for solace, and pencil and paper became my means of self-discovery. I drew in silence and allowed whatever was in my mind to take form and flow out. There was no conscious creation, just flow.

At that time, I knew nothing of my direction. I let go of expectation, and that was when a kind, compassionate, loving man came into my life. It was not something I expected or sought, but help was nonetheless welcome.

Then the real work began. All those issues I thought I had expertly evaded stepped neatly into my path. I learned the only way out of this was through it. I could continue sitting in the muck and crying over all the injustice, or I could pick myself up and walk toward something that fed me rather than fed *on* me. I did not know where I was going, but anywhere was better than where I had been stuck for many years.

I learned that balance is not static. Life is fluid. The more rigidity in my thoughts, muscles, spirit, or emotions, the harder life became. At each transition, no matter how much I cried, screamed, or whined, the only way out was to step into action.

I am still learning these lessons at different levels today. Once I think I have it wrangled, another layer of understanding opens. The more I learn, the more I know the minuteness of my understanding. The truth is, we are all perpetual beginners. Each moment is new with opportunities that may not have been present before. These realizations broadened my horizons and made things I never fathomed a possibility. Over time, these possibilities became my new reality.

I began experiencing moments of lightness, moments where the flow of life and I were in unison. At first, these moments flitted in and out with little rhyme or reason. As I evolved and let go of needing to be in control, the moments became more frequent and lasted longer. Now I am quicker to notice when I stray from my path. It is easier to center and ground myself each time I step forward on new terrain toward my goals. Healing, health, life, success, and love are not linear. That was a delusion I had labored under, but these things just don't move in a straight line.

I learned that if I don't value and understand myself, no one would be able to truly care for or understand me fully. Caring for and loving myself gave me more tools to help others. As I learned to pay attention to my reactions and rhythms, I saw that our cycles and those of nature are intrinsically linked. All the pain, impulses, and desires were telling me the answers to the big questions of life. What am I hungry for? What do I want out of life?

Through personal study, I found herbs, food, and hydrotherapy methods that helped me feel better and lessened my pain. This love of herbs and nutrition lead me to work with naturopaths, counsellors, and acupuncturists.

I wanted to help others understand that they too could take charge of their health. I earned my Doctorate of Naturopathic Medicine at Bastyr University, where I studied for five years. I explored advanced homeopathy at the New England School of

Homeopathy, and extended my knowledge through the guidance of teachers at National College of Naturopathic Medicine. Dr. Dickson Thom (DDS, ND) was particularly influential.

Ghandi said it well: "Be the change you wish to see in the world." I take this to heart. I have lost many amazing people in my life, in many different ways, but they taught me to seize the moment, be true to myself, and say what I need to say because sometimes one chance is all I have.

So love it up. Own yourself and your actions. Be patient with your imperfections; they may one day be powerful assets. Be aware of limiting excuses about why you cannot live fully at this moment. Excuses are the lies of the frightened. I know; I was once frightened myself.

Take a calculated risk and find out who you truly are; you are definitely worth knowing.

1

Nourishing Space Within:

Get the Most Out of This Book

Just when the caterpillar thought the world was over, it became a butterfly.

~Proverb

Self-care is not something we were all taught as children. Most of us were taught to brush our teeth, go to bed at a certain hour, and eat three meals a day. Self-care is larger than these basics and extends to caring for your mind, body, and spirit.

This book is intended to help you build your available resources and form daily habits that can support your health and happiness throughout life, no matter the conditions and situations you find yourself facing.

Your most valuable resource is your health, and self-care is a powerful tool for preserving it. When you choose to give yourself the gift of self-care, you allow yourself to experience life with greater ease and grace. No one can do it for you; you are the only one who can take care of your core self at this level.

The more consistent you are with your self-care, the more benefit you can be to others. By caring for yourself, you give others permission to care about themselves. They too will understand that it is okay to take the time and create space to care for oneself. If you wish to build a healthy world, you must start within.

There are many benefits to committing to a regular self-care routine. Learning to listen to the messages your body is giving you provides opportunity to deal with health issues before they blow up and create serious, long-term damage. Self-care also helps you create more space within, allowing more room for you to grow and relax into your true self.

The simple and effective self-care techniques I have included in this book are not new. They are a collection of naturopathic techniques and traditional self-care methods designed to support health—physical, mental, emotional, and spiritual. I became familiar with these techniques while in naturopathic school and through my extended education. Together, we will explore many different ways to help your mind, body, and spirit work as efficiently and effortlessly as possible.

I recommend variants of these self-care tools to patients of all ages. In my practice I see that a majority of my patients who apply these tools consistently get better faster and with less aggra-vation. Their minds begin to calm. Better nourishing choices are made with ease and they enjoy their everyday lives more and rely less on willpower to get the daily routines done.

Understanding yourself is not an easy task. Our society is not built to support this awareness. The better you understand your-self, the more clearly you will see the world around you and the less likely you will be to accept and support injustice.

While this path is not an easy one, it is more than worth every single step toward a better you. One step at a time is the only way to get anywhere. Each step gets easier and picks up momen-tum. "One breath at a time" was the mantra that helped me in difficult times. It reminded me that I did not have to, nor could I, change everything all at once. The knowledge that each breath is a new beginning helped me keep things in perspective.

Setbacks and obstacles are not there to hinder and hurt you; they teach you how to achieve your goal and give you tools you need to attain it. If you never fell short or "failed," how could you improve skills, reactions, or thoughts? So when you fall down, go ahead and cry, kick, scream, and wallow. Get it out. Then get back up and keep going. The journey is where all the great stories and memories are waiting to bless you. Just remember to breathe.

We are our own jailers. But the keys to unlocking the bonds that imprison us lie within the bonds themselves. Know that when seeking to change yourself, your ego will rebel and resistance will arise. This resistance may take many forms: excuses, illness in yourself or others, stress, tears, tantrums, loved ones nay-saying, and an amazing zest for all the little chores that were once put on the back burner that suddenly need to be done now. These obstacles will present themselves when you initiate change, and again when you are on the doorstep of your dreams.

Remember that resistance gives you a chance to practice and show your commitment to your goals. Be patient, take a deep breath, and *keep going*. Understanding your resistance changes the way you interact with yourself at a core level and allows the good stuff to settle in and put down roots.

If you are truly invested in change, you will find the time and resources for self-care, but support of some kind is indispensable on this path. Counselors, acupuncturists, homeopaths, compassionate, positive friends, and, of course, naturopathic doctors are great resources to help you objectively assess and address obstacles that arise.

To avoid feeling overwhelmed, I invite you to pick one or two techniques or changes that resonate with you and make you excited. Tuck them into your schedule and do them at the same time every day. Let technology support you with reminders on your phone to help you create a habit. Take baby steps, and when those first changes begin to feel easy and normal, consider adding others, one by one.

Allow yourself to enjoy the adventure of getting to know your self with curiosity and compassion. Soon you will find your lost rhythm. Soon you will fall into step with the pace of nature. Soon you will thrive.

Don't wait!

2

Naturopathic Medicine:

An Overview

You never change things by fighting the existing reality. To change something, build a new model that makes the existing model obsolete.

~Buckminster Fuller

Naturopathic medicine has a broad scope and uses many different approaches and modalities. As with all medicine, but showing up strongly in naturopathic medicine, each physician applies her own personal understanding to her knowledge of healing. The core philosophies that guide this understanding and unite all naturopathic physicians allow us to tailor treatments to each individual.

This is my understanding of the six tenets of naturopathic medicine:

1. **First, do no harm:** As a naturopathic doctor, I use the least invasive and most effective treatment possible, considering the short and long-term affects of each recommendation given.

2. **Identify and treat the cause**: Symptoms are the body's way of letting us know something is out of balance. I treat the symptom and the underlying cause of the symptom, thereby helping patients heal at a deeper level. If I treat the symptom only, I fail to restore true wholeness and health. If the symptom is only covered up or suppressed and not treated at the core level, it will return in another form.

3. **Treat the whole person**: The physical, mental, emotional, and spiritual aspects of each patient's life play a role in the journey toward wellness. I take all these aspects into account in order to create the most effective treatments.

4. **The body has innate ability to heal**: Our bodies know how to heal. Yet, when we are overwhelmed with toxins and stress, our systems cannot function smoothly and properly. I help patients learn to identify and address the obstacles to healing while moving toward optimal health.

5. **Doctor as teacher:** My goal is to practice, teach, inspire, and empower my patients to choose healthy lifestyles. These choices are the foundation of health. Life, with

its many twists and turns, affects the way we feel in our bodies and I aim to help patients meet obstacles gracefully.

6. **Prevention is cure:** Prevention is more effective and less expensive than treating a disease. I seek to reduce imbalances, which could, if left unaddressed, lead to degenerative diseases.

Optimizing Emunctories:

Opening the Doors

When you follow your bliss . . . doors will open where there were no doors before, where you would not have thought there were going to be doors, and where there wouldn't be a door for anyone else.

~Joseph Campbell

Your major organs of elimination are called emunctories. The primary emunctories are skin, lungs, colon, and kidneys. Your emotions are your energetic emunctory.

Your body has an innate ability to release toxins through your emunctories, and this release is necessary for healing. Unfortunately, during times of stress, your ability to eliminate waste and toxins closes down. Conscious support is needed to open and maintain the function of these doors.

When your emunctories are closed, little can get out, and it is difficult to truly heal. In this blocked state, your body needs to put waste from normal metabolic functions—breathing, digestion, and movement—somewhere. It tucks these waste products into your tissues, causing pain and inflammation.

Imagine you are a cup. All the things in your everyday life that you process, such as food, information, external toxins, and emotional experiences, are water that fills the cup. In times of stress, more water trickles into the cup. Extra stressors, such as deadline-oriented work, driving in traffic, exposure to pesticides, and dealing with emotional trauma, are extra portions of water. The cup soon fills up, and if your body is to continue to function and allow you to process new input, water must also move out of the cup.

Imagine there are a few small holes around the base of your cup, each allowing a little water to flow out. These holes represent your organs of elimination. Your enzyme systems, hormone balance, and stress management tools help break down stressors so they are easier to eliminate. But when constant stress affects these systems, debris can build up. Blockages can clog the little holes at the base of your cup.

Physically, you may begin to show symptoms, and you may shut down emotionally or become hyper-reactive. As stressors keep coming, your cup continues to fill. If the parade of insults continues, soon your cup is close to overflowing. In this state, even minor stressors can compromise your ability to eliminate, leaving you in a more reactive and defensive state.

Cultivating self-care in your life allows your organs of elimination to begin to reopen the blocked holes at the base of your cup, allowing your system to flow properly again.

In this chapter, I will describe simple and effective ways to support the opening and balanced function of your emunctories. Following these guidelines will help your body eliminate what no longer serves you. When you are open and in the flow, endless possibilities open before you.

Lungs

Your lungs take care of gas exchange. Every cell in your body makes carbon dioxide as a waste product. If you are not breathing fully, you are not fully eliminating this waste. When carbon dioxide builds up in your tissues, you become more inflamed, acidic, and reactive both physically and emotionally. The best way to support your lungs is with deep breathing.

Create space with breath work

Focusing on your breath is a simple place to start and, over time, helps quiet the noise in your mind. Noise will always be around, waiting to rush in and fill your mind. In the beginning, it may help to choose quiet locations for this work to diminish interruptions, but you may eventually find that you can incorporate breath exercises into your daily routine.

Often when you quiet your surroundings, internal dialogue seems amplified. This is normal, and part of normal resistance. Noise will diminish with practice, but it will never go away completely. Try not to judge what comes up in the silence. Acknowledge it, then let it go and return awareness to your breath. Don't worry; you will have infinite opportunities to practice this new pattern. Remember that the benefit lies in the practice, not in achieving perfection.

Cultivating internal quiet is where transformation begins. Here I offer different meditation and breathing techniques to help nourish your internal space. I recommend starting with five to 10 minutes a day of focused breath work and then work up to work up to 30 minutes, or even an hour if you are truly inspired by the changes you begin to notice. Feel free to break it up into smaller portions, or go for one longer session. If time is limited, do your breathing exercises while you are doing other chores such as laundry, dishes, or showering.

Exercise: Basic Deep Abdominal Breaths

This exercise can be done standing, seated, or lying down. Begin where you're most comfortable.

Start by inhaling slowly through your nose. Be aware of your shoulders: keep them level, down, and back. As you inhale, allow your abdomen to expand. While learning, it helps to put your hands over your belly to engage this motion fully. Upon your exhale, breathe out through your mouth like you're blowing through a straw. While you exhale, draw your abdomen back toward your spine.

Be aware of what the air feels like as it fills your lungs and again as it exits your body. Try to make your exhale slightly longer than your inhale. This helps to release more carbon dioxide. The goal is slow, smooth, steady and silent.

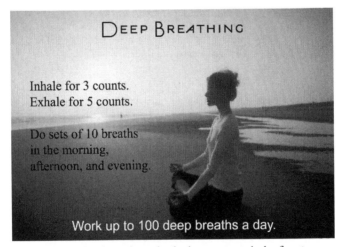

DEEP BREATHING

Inhale for 3 counts.
Exhale for 5 counts.

Do sets of 10 breaths
in the morning,
afternoon, and evening.

Work up to 100 deep breaths a day.

Try the basic rhythm described above, or inhale for 1 count, hold for 4 counts, exhale for 2 counts.

Variations

You can amplify the effects of breath work by adding visualizations. Inhaling what you want—love, patience, serenity, or restful sleep—and exhaling what no longer serves you—fear, jealousy, anger, judgment, or tension.

Another option is to imagine inhaling a color or image you find soothing. Then imagine exhaling a color or image signifying what you no longer wish to carry.

I recommend integrating 100 conscious deep breaths into your day. Many people find putting notes in prominent places helpful in creating this habit. Put them on your mirror, fridge, steering wheel, computer, anywhere you look frequently, or set reminders on your cell phone. With regular practice, you will find your breaths becoming steadier, deeper and less labored.

❋ Exercise: Zen Breath Counting

This is a good exercise if you need to focus on something more than just your breath. Practice the Basic Deep Abdominal Breaths from above, counting each breath. The goal is to count up to 25 breaths without other thoughts running through your mind. If a thought does pop up, acknowledge it without judgment and let it go, then start back counting again at one. This helps to cultivate focus and clarity.

This one always makes me laugh. I inevitably count to the early teens and then I think "Hey, great! I'm doing it! Oh, wait. Nope....One...." This technique helped me be less judgmental of my thoughts, and in turn, less judgmental of others.

Lymph

The lymphatic system is your body's garbage collector. If the lymphatic system is not working, it is difficult for all your other systems to function properly. It's like trying to live in your house without taking out the garbage. Things would get stinky, toxic, and the functionality of your house would diminish as the rooms fill up with waste.

The lymphatic system is a network of fluid, vessels, and nodes. The nodes are the easiest to identify, as they tend to swell when you are ill. You may have noticed when you get a cold that the nodes under your jaw become swollen and tender to touch. The lymph nodes are located along the vessels and serve as check points looking for pathogens. When pathogens are identified, the node swells, trapping them. The immune system is then called in to deal with them appropriately.

The lymphatic vessels run just under the skin carrying lymphatic fluid upward toward the heart. They don't have valves, so they rely on support from deep breathing and muscular movement to drain. There are other ways we can support and bolster lymphatic function, including castor oil packs, dry skin brushing, QiGong, Tai Chi, rebounding, and lymphatic massage.

❋ Exercise: Castor Oil Packs

Castor oil packs are the most important thing you can do to support your lymphatic health. Castor oil is a vegetable oil drawn from the seed of the castor oil plant.

Castor oil packs aid in elimination and detoxification processes in the body, through a mechanism likely related to its numbing and anti-inflammatory properties. It has a variety of uses for health, but in the naturopathic model, castor oil is applied topically to increase lymphatic fluid movement, support waste collection and elimination, and draw white blood cells to the area where it is applied. White blood cells are your patrols helping to locate and eliminate pathogens. Another benefit of castor oil is its affinity with the nervous system, helping to increase calm and balance.[i]

This is one of my favorite personal experiences with the versatility of castor oil. At our last home we had chickens. One got out and wandered into a stand of olive trees to forage. She got spooked, wedged herself into the thorny branches, and was distressed to the point I felt I only had time to grab gloves before I headed in after her. Needless to say, extracting a frightened hen from an olive tree densely covered with 2-inch thorns left me with deep scratches up and down my arms.

After the hen was safely back with her friends, I washed my arms and gently pressed castor oil into the scratches. I applied the oil a few times a day. After one day, the scratches were 50 per cent better and almost totally cleared within three days.

CASTOR OIL PACKS
Key to lymphatic health.

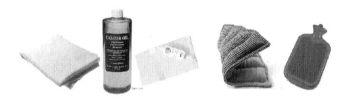

Castor oil packs are supportive for many different issues such as uterine fibroids, benign ovarian cysts, headaches, liver disorders, abdominal pain, constipation, diarrhea, intestinal disorders, gallbladder inflammation or stones, night time urinary frequency, and inflamed joints. Consult your physician before using castor oil packs during pregnancy, active ulcers, or if you have bleeding disorders.

You can find castor oil at most natural food stores or in pharmacies. Look for cold-pressed and ideally organic versions. Results are cumulative and best when the pack is applied nightly or at least four nights in a row each week.

Supplies:
- Clean, dry flannel cloth or hand towel, made of cotton or wool (20" to 40" x 24" to 48")
- Hot water bottle or heating pack made of flax, rice, or gel
- Castor oil
- One or two old, large towels

- Blanket
- Large plastic bag with zipper closure

Directions:

1. Fold the cloth so that it fits over your entire abdomen. If there are breast or lung issues, the cloth will need to cover the entire chest and abdomen.

2. Lay down in a comfortable position on an old towel with all your supplies near you. The towel will prevent staining your bed. Castor oil stains are difficult to remove, so be cautious.

3. Drizzle 1 or 2 tablespoons of castor oil on the cloth. Fold cloth in half to disperse the oil, then unfold and apply to abdomen and/or chest. Cover castor oil cloth with an old towel.

   Note that in the first couple of weeks, you may need to add an additional tablespoon of oil every few days. Eventually, the cloth will be saturated enough that reapplication of oil will only be needed every couple of weeks. The cloth should not be dripping. It should have just enough oil, so if you were to touch the compress to a piece of wood, it would polish the wood with no drips or runs.

4. Place a heating pack over the towel. Cover yourself with a warm blanket.

5. Leave the castor oil pack on for 30 to 60 minutes. This is an excellent time to practice your breathing exercises, visualization, or meditation. Individuals with chemical sensitivity disorders may have more symptoms after using the castor oil pack, especially at the beginning of treatment, since it stimulates the process of elimination and detoxification. If this is true for you, start with only five minutes a day and slowly increase over time.

6. It is fine to fall asleep with the castor oil pack on, as long as you are not using an electrical heating source.

7. When done, you may leave oil on the skin to completely absorb, or remove the oil with a solution of 2 tablespoons baking soda to 1 quart of water, or hair conditioner applied alone works well. There should be only a thin layer of oil left on the skin after the pack.

8. When you are done, store the pack in a large plastic bag with an air-tight closure. The castor oil pack can be used repeatedly. If the smell or color changes, dispose of the pack and create another.

Skin

Your skin eliminates through sweat. When its ability to release toxins is overwhelmed, the skin begins to show irritation, which may manifest as itching, rashes, acne, rosacea, boils, or hives, to name a few.

✳ Exercise: Dry Skin Brushing

You can support your skin by dry skin brushing. This practice removes dead skin cells and stimulates blood and lymph flow to the skin, enabling the skin's ability to release toxins from your body.

The best skin brushes are natural vegetable bristle brushes. You can find these brushes in most health food stores. If the bristles are too stiff for you, start with a natural loofah. Once your skin is stronger and better conditioned, shift to the natural vegetable bristle brush.

Skin brushing is best done on dry skin, prior to bed or your shower or bath. Brushing should be gentle, and done in short strokes toward the heart. This is because dry skin brushing also has the benefit of encouraging lymphatic flow, and lymphatic fluid always drains toward the heart.

DRY SKIN BRUSHING

With a stiff-bristled brush,
apply short and brisk
strokes toward the heart.

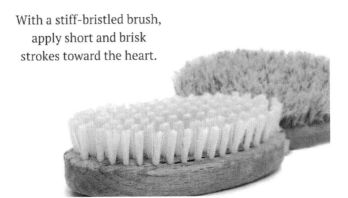

Directions:

1. Start by brushing your legs. Brush in small strokes from your toes, remembering to brush your soles. Slowly move up your legs towards the center of your body. This motion should not be aggressive, but more like you are petting yourself. When finished, your skin will tingle and might be a little red, but if your skin is bright red you are brushing too hard.

2. Next, brush lightly up your stomach and lower back, making sure to include your buttocks. Always move toward your heart.

3. Move to your arms and brush from your fingers to your shoulders in short strokes toward the center of your body.

4. Lightly brush your shoulders and upper back toward your armpits.

5. Your breasts should be brushed from the nipple outward, like the spokes of a wheel.

6. Do not brush your face, as this skin is very delicate. However, you can lightly brush down the back of your neck.

Please avoid the following areas: Open wounds, your face, areas of skin that are easily damaged, areas of known skin malignancies or lymphatic malignancies, and open and weeping rashes.

Kidneys

Your kidneys filter blood and lymphatic fluid, separating out liquid waste. It is fitting that fluids support your kidneys' ability to filter and function, but not all fluids are supportive. Water, herbal tea, broth, kombucha, kefir (water or milk), and raw milk are nourishing and hydrating, while caffeinated beverages such as coffee, black and green teas, soda, energy drinks, and juice and alcohol are dehydrating and do not support the kidneys. If you do choose to drink these, add an additional cup of water to your day.

Fluid intake is not one-size-fits-all. In general, a good goal is consuming about half your weight in ounces. So if you weigh about 150 pounds, your goal is to drink 75 ounces (about 9.5 cups) of hydrating fluids a day. Don't like drinking water? Add a little fresh squeezed lemon or lime juice, or a pinch of unrefined sea salt (one with lots of color for more trace minerals) to your water to aid assimilation and balance electrolytes. Herbal teas are another great option and can be enjoyed iced or hot.

Sipping water throughout the day supports elimination and fluid balance. I recommend finding a water bottle you enjoying looking at so you're more prone to pick it up and drink. I like non-leaching stainless-steel bottles for their strength and durability.

Colon

Your colon takes care of solid waste disposal. It is also the seat of 70 per cent of your immune system.[ii]

Bacterial balance greatly influences colon and immune function. There are 10 times more bacterial cells in and on us than there are human cells.[iii] It is important to support the good bacteria, also called "probiotics," because they live symbiotically with us, unlike pathogenic bacteria.

When the bacterial balance in your gut is thrown off, you may experience abdominal pain, gas, bloating, constipation, diarrhea, headaches, anxiety, depression, frequent infections, obesity, and immune deficiencies. The delicate balance is disrupted by antibiotics, stress, hormone imbalances, and processed foods such as flours, oils, sugars, and genetically modified organisms (GMOs).

The best way to support the colon is with fermented foods. These foods trump any probiotic supplement with greater bacterial diversity than any pill could offer. Be cautious with probiotic supplements. Often they have different strains or volume of organisms than stated on the packaging. Make sure you find a reputable brand with third-party testing if you choose to use a supplement. Better yet, let food be your medicine.

4

Food:

Nourishing Our Bodies

*Let food be thy medicine and
medicine be thy food.*

~Hippocrates

What is a healthy diet? This is a huge question and there is much confusion and misinformation everywhere you look. This chapter provides some basic guidelines for increasing the nutrient density of your diet.

Let me start by explaining that the word diet has a bad reputation and is often associated with deprivation. When I use the word diet, I am talking about the foods you habitually eat, both good and bad. The more naturally occurring nutrients you can get in your diet, the stronger your body, mind, and spirit.

Our country is one of the most affluent countries in the world, yet it has the highest rates of chronic disease. In our country, food is degraded, stripped of its nutrients, synthetically fortified, and presented as "whole" food. Food preparation has been removed from the home and given to corporations. Some people spend huge amounts of money to buy prepared foods made with cheap, low-quality ingredients. They may also buy vitamin supplements to fill the nutrient gap in their diets, pushing the cost of eating processed food even higher.

What is the cost of trading convenience for quality? Rates of diabetes are skyrocketing and it is now estimated over one third of our population will be diabetic within the next 20 years[iv]. Obesity, chronic diseases and infections are rampant in our society. Food allergies and sensitivities, autism[v], attention deficit disorder, attention deficit hyperactivity, cancer; all of these are increasing at a shocking rate.

Why are we so sick, tired, and broken down in our society? Something is not working.

As I began to study nutrition privately and in school, modern approaches to food seemed overly complicated and complex. I could not wrap my head around why vegetable oils and other modern inventions were considered healthier than fats humans had used for centuries. Foods we evolved eating, such as butter and lard, had been transformed into villains over a period of about 100 years.

Things began to make sense in my mind when a mentor introduced me to the work of Dr. Weston A. Price. Price was an American dentist who investigated traditional diets. Working in the early 1900s, he noticed his patients had increasing numbers of cavities, more incidences of crooked teeth, and more palate deformities. He watched the community around him become more ill. He began to wonder if food was the culprit.

Price had heard stories about people with straight, white teeth in faraway primitive tribes. He wanted to find out what these people ate, and if the rumors were true about their health. So he and his wife packed up their lives and traveled around the world seeking isolated tribes in Switzerland, the Outer Hebrides, North America, Malaysia, Polynesia, Africa, Australia, New Zealand, and South America.

These isolated groups of people did not trade for commodities such as flour, sugar, and canned goods because their locations were remote. They consumed grown, foraged, or hunted food from their local areas. Price interviewed these people, took pictures, and brought samples of their food back to his labs to test their nutrient value. He compared their diets with dietary information gathered from people in nearby cities.

Price found nearly perfect dental health in these isolated tribes, who were also generally healthier than their urban counterparts. The isolated groups did not have the modern diseases of headaches, fatigue, cardiovascular disease, fertility issues, or cancer. Even the eldest members were strong, active, and quick witted.

Price's data showed that diets from the isolated tribes, while there was tremendous variation in what they ate, had consistent similarities. He found no processed foods. All groups ate some type of animal products, and if large animals were eaten, organ meats were highly prized. Price found no vegan societies. Their foods were nutrient dense and had much higher levels of fat-soluble vitamins (Vitamin A, D, E, and K) than similar food found in nearby cities. Every group had some kind of enzyme-rich food made by fermentation or culturing. Everything was seasonal. Grains, seeds, legumes were always soaked, fermented, or sprouted. One of his biggest surprises was the level of fat intake. The tribes he studied consumed high fat diets and they mainly consumed saturated fats such as tallow, lard, butter, palm, seal oil, and whale oil.

When members of the isolated groups began to travel and eat modern foods they began experiencing these modern diseases including increasing rates of cavities. Their children, first generation modern food consumers, began to show physical defects, crooked teeth, and other developmental disorders. This effect occurs even today with immigrants who adopt the standard American diet. Chronic diseases are close on the heels of these food changes.

I teach nutrition classes in my town and have done so for years. In these classes, I advise a diet similar to the one Price described. My students are often shocked to realize how far a standard American diet is from healthy. Sometimes I can see my students becoming overwhelmed as we discuss the differences and how they might make positive changes. I emphasize that each small change is a victory. All that matters is that these changes are sustainable.

What does this dietary approach mean to you in a modern urban environment where convenient and prepared foods are the norm? The answer is simple. Get back to basics. The goal is just eat *real* food.

♠ Food Tool: What is Real Food?

Some good questions to ask yourself
- Is the ingredient list long enough to be a book?
- Does it have acronyms, numbers, chemicals, or lab-created ingredients?
- Do I know what the words mean?
- Do I use these ingredients in my kitchen?
- Have we been eating this food in this form for thousands of years?

- If I point to the food on my plate, is it recognizable for what it is?

The more processed your food, even in your own kitchen, the further it gets from its natural state. If you see an ingredient list that looks like a novel with acronyms, chemical names, and unpronounceable words, that food might not be the best choice. Choose foods with simple ingredients that you would use in your kitchen. Better yet, make it yourself.

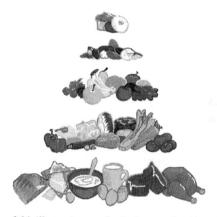

At the top of this illustration, see foods that you should eat in extreme moderation. At the bottom, see foods you should enjoy frequently.

Diet Basics

While I tailor diets to each individual in my practice, here is a tool that will help you know what to include and what to avoid when building a nutrient-dense diet.

♠ Food Tool: Diet Basics to Enjoy, Limit, Avoid

Foods to enjoy frequently

- Pasture-raised or wild meat and eggs

- Raw, whole-fat dairy

- Local, seasonal vegetables, and fruits

- Quality fats, such as butter, olive oil, lard, tallow, and coconut oil

- Whole grains (minimal amounts, if tolerated)
- Fermented foods such as kefir (water or milk), cheese, sauerkraut, kimchi, kombucha, yogurt
- Grains, nuts, and legumes that have been soaked, fermented, or sprouted
- Clean water
- Unrefined sea salt

Foods to avoid or limit
- Processed cereals, such as packaged cereals, granola bars, and protein bars
- Conventionally raised meat, dairy, and eggs
- Refined sugar
- White flours
- Vegetable oils
- Corn syrup (all kinds)
- Ultra-pasteurized dairy
- Processed foods
- Canned foods (look instead for foods preserved in glass)
- Preservatives
- Artificial sweeteners

Do the best you can. Making changes to your diet is not all-or-nothing. At the same time, be honest with yourself about your relationship with food and why you make your food choices.

I like the 80/20 approach. Do your best at home with 80 per cent of your meals. If you can afford to eat out, you can afford to buy better quality food for home consumption. Allow some wiggle room for the remaining 20 per cent of food purchased, unless food allergies or intolerances are present. By cleaning up your diet, you gain a clearer view of where your personal food boundaries are and where you can be flexible.

Prioritize to stay on budget

Most of us are on a budget and must be conscientious about how we spend our food dollars. We also want to make sure to use every part of our food possible to minimize waste. For example, try conserving chicken bones or leftover vegetables to make nutritious broths.

The tools below will help you determine where to focus your funds and where you have wiggle room. Choose items from the top of the following best-to-worst lists whenever possible.

♠ Food Tool: Choosing Fruit, Grains, Legumes, Nuts, Seeds, Vegetables

In order from best to worst
- Biodynamic* and local
- Biodynamic
- Organic and local
- Organic
- Conventional and local
- Conventional**

*Biodynamic is a method of organic farming that cultivates the development and collaboration of soil, plants, and animals into a self-sustaining system

**Eating real food, even conventionally grown and raised, removes a lot of extra faux foods. Even if you cannot afford organic, removing processed versions of flour, dairy, meat, and sugar, as well as, canned foods, would be a nutritional advantage.

Growing your own food is a cheap and easy way to boost your nutrition. If you have a lawn, consider converting part of it into a garden. If you don't have a lawn, a window box of herbs is a great option. Fresh herbs are simple and help boost flavor and nutrient density.

All fruits and vegetables are best consumed fresh and seasonally. If needed, preserve the season's bounty by fermentation, freezing, or drying in order to retain as much of the nutrient density as possible.

♠ Food Tool: Choosing Meat, Eggs, Dairy

In order from best to worst

- Wild
- Grass-fed and grass-finished
- Grass-fed and grain-finished
- Organic
- Conventional is not recommended

Animal products such as meat, milk, and eggs are the most important items to choose wisely. Happy animals are raised outside and forage for what they want to eat. These animals are optimal for your health and the environment. There more omega-3, CLA, and vitamins D and A in animals that are raised outside and have the option to eat what they desire. Happy animals translate to meat, eggs, and dairy that nourish and decrease inflammation rather than perpetuate it.

When buying meat, purchase meat with the bone in, and save the bones for broth. Ask the butcher to cut the bones into 2- to 4-inch pieces to make them easier for you to use at home.

Buying in bulk is much more cost effective. Go in with your friends to get the best deal on locally raised meat to extend your buying power.

Make sure to include organ meats and bones in your order. Organ meats are cheap and highly nutritious. These are great extenders of ground meat and do not affect flavor when used in small amounts. For example, mixing minced liver into ground meat for meatloaf is a good start. Start small by adding a ground teaspoon per pound, and slowly increase the amount.

When choosing animals raised for consumption, make sure you know what they were fed. Ask questions and get to know your farmer. Genetically modified organisms (GMOs) and the pesticides applied to vegetables and grains are compounded in conventionally raised animals.

Genetically Modified Organisms

Genetically modified organisms (GMOs) are foods altered by removing genes or adding foreign virus, bacteria, or genetic material into plants and animals. GMOs are associated with infertility, immunity problems, accelerated aging, diabetes, cancer, increased sensitivity to foods, and have a greater negative impact on children, pregnant women, and the elderly.[vi]

Some foods are GMO unless they are specified organic or non-GMO, including corn, soy, canola, cottonseed, sugar from sugar beets, Hawaiian papaya, crookneck squash, some zucchinis, potatoes, tomatoes, and chocolate.[vii] It is not necessary to completely remove these foods. Choosing organic versions will greatly decrease your GMO intake. This is a big step, requiring commitment and vigilance.

Unfortunately, our general food supply is no longer trustworthy. You can change this by being aware of where you spend your money. If you choose wisely where to spend your dollars, you can change the market and the world.

Pesticides

Most conventional pesticides kill insects by damaging their nervous system. Unfortunately, this affects your nervous system too. Pesticide exposure happens in many different ways. The most common exposures are through eating conventionally sprayed produce, and by eating meat from animals raised in confined feedlots, since their food is contaminated. If you live in an agricultural area, you could be exposed to drift from sprayed pesticides as well as contaminated well water.

Organic gardening practices help nourish the soil and provide more nutrient-dense foods. If the soil is not healthy and full of nutrients, it will not produce healthy food. In a global sense, pesticides affect far more than the crops treated directly. Pesticides and fertilizers threaten the health of farm workers. They wash down through the soil and into the aquifer, where they travel into your water supply, tainting your drinking water. They also flush into rivers and streams, then into the ocean, which affects sea vegetables and the fish we consume, creating a cascade of damaging effects worldwide.

Reducing pesticide exposure

Sometimes the cost of organic produce can be prohibitive. Keep in mind that not all foods are sprayed equally. The Environmental Working Group looked at residual pesticide levels on vegetables and fruits after they are rinsed with water, the washing method most of us use at home. The most contaminated foods have been dubbed the "Dirty Dozen Plus" and the least contaminated are known as the "Clean Fifteen." Pesticide-laden foods are listed below in order of contamination. The most contaminated are ideally eaten organic or avoided.

♠ Food Tool: Dirty Dozen Plus[viii]

Top 12 most pesticide-laden foods, in order of contamination

1. Apples
2. Peaches
3. Nectarines
4. Strawberries
5. Grapes
6. Celery
7. Spinach
8. Sweet bell peppers
9. Cucumbers
10. Cherry tomatoes
11. Snap peas (imported)
12. Potatoes
13. Hot peppers
14. Kale/Collard greens

Then there are the Clean Fifteen. These are foods that do not need to be purchased organic, as the pesticide levels found are relatively low.

♠ Food Tool: Clean Fifteen

Top 15 cleanest foods, in order of purity
1. Avocado
2. Sweet corn (most likely GMO, so choose organic)
3. Pineapple
4. Cabbage
5. Sweet peas (frozen)
6. Onions
7. Asparagus
8. Mango
9. Papaya (most likely GMO, so choose organic if it is from Hawaii*)
10. Kiwi
11. Eggplant
12. Grapefruit
13. Cantaloupe
14. Cauliflower
15. Sweet potatoes

This 2015 information is provided annually by the Environmental Working Group, ewg.org.

*GMO laws in Hawaii are changing but there are loopholes for existing farms.

Salt

Salt is the only rock we eat. It is such an important mineralized rock that people used to be paid in salt, hence the origin of the word "salary." As with many ancient foods, salt is currently misunderstood. It is the processing and excessive consumption of salt—not salt itself—that contributes to high blood pressure, stroke, and even osteoporosis. But does that mean you must drastically reduce your salt intake in order to be healthy? I think it is more important to look at the quality of the salt we consume.

Avoid pure, white table salt. The processing this salt undergoes rips out minerals and adds anti-caking agents such as sodium silicoaluminate. Table salt is the number one source of aluminum in the American diet, causing oxidative damage to brain tissues.[ix] Eliminating or decreasing processed and boxed foods reduces the amount of processed sale you consume.

Whole, real salt is colorful. Color indicates the presence of trace minerals. This is the kind of salt to choose. Your body needs salt for protein and carbohydrate digestion. Salt is a major electrolyte that helps you maintain proper hydration. Your adrenal glands use salt to function properly. Salt is mandatory for basic cellular metabolism throughout the body.

Iodized salt is commonly available in stores, and while iodine is important in the diet, it is better to get it from whole foods than from processed salt. Iodine-rich foods include wild fish, sea vegetables (seaweed, kombu, wakame), pastured eggs, pastured butter and milk. Please keep in mind that for animal products to be rich in iodine, they must be raised on iodine-rich soil. This is why it is important to know where your food comes from.

In the store, look for salt that is colorful (gray, red or pink) and has visible signs of moisture; these are all hallmarks of quality unrefined sea salt. Some salts are more nutrient dense than others. Celtic sea salt has one of the highest mineral contents. While greater nutritional density is not an excuse to salt your food heavily, increasing the quality of food, including salt, in your diet can increase your health.

Buying in bulk is a great way to decrease the cost of quality ingredients, so talk with friends about sharing larger quantities.

Fats

Quality fat is very important. Price found the isolated tribes he studied consumed an average of 40 to 70 per cent fat. The quality and type of fat is the key. Examples of these healthy fats are butter, olive oil, lard, tallow, and coconut oil. In the early 1900s, Americans, on average, consumed about 18 pounds of butter a year. Now vegetable oils (corn, canola, cottonseed, safflower, and soy oils) are the primary fats in our modern diet.

There are many reasons you need good fat in your diet. Good fat is essential to health. Every cell in the body is protected by membranes made of fat, half of which is saturated. In order for your cells to function properly they must have healthy and flexible cell boundaries.

Hormones are made with fat, with the backbone of all hormones coming from cholesterol. Increasing good fat intake can help improve your mood and even help you lose weight. If you don't have enough good fat, your metabolism and endocrine system don't have the building blocks they need to make healthy amounts of hormones that maintain balance. Hormones regulate sleep, menstrual cycles, mood, weight, and many other functions of your body.

Fat and the vitamins it carries are paramount for proper immune function. Fat-soluble vitamins are D, A, K, and E.

♠ Food Tool: Fats to Enjoy, Limit, Avoid

Fats to enjoy frequently
- Butter from pasture-raised cows, goats, and sheep
- Chicken, duck, and goose fat from pasture-raised poultry
- Cold-pressed coconut oil
- Cold-pressed cod liver oil
- Cold-pressed flax oil (freshly pressed, eaten raw and kept refrigerated)
- Cold-pressed olive oil (ideally raw)

- Cold-pressed sesame oil
- Fish (wild)
- Lard from pasture-raised pigs
- Tallow from pasture-raised beef and lamb

Fats to limit
- Peanut oil
- Sunflower seed oil

Fats to avoid
- Hydrogenated and partially hydrogenated oils (trans-fats)
- Margarine
- Shortening
- Vegetable oils (including corn, soy, canola/rapeseed, cottonseed, safflower)

Dairy

Dairy is ideal when raw. In its raw form, it is packed with beneficial enzymes and is a living food. Among other enzymes, raw milk contains lactase, an enzyme that helps break down lactose, the sugar in dairy that causes many people to become sensitive to milk. Lactase is damaged in the pasteurization process, as are B vitamins.

Reduced-fat milk and ultra-pasteurized dairy are no longer whole foods. Ultra-pasteurization oxidizes the cholesterol in the milk, making it highly inflammatory.

♠ Food Tool: Types of Dairy

In order of intact beneficial nutrients
- Raw
- Vat pasteurized
- Pasteurized
- Ultra-pasteurized (avoid)

Fish

The benefits of eating seafood outweigh the current negative side effects from toxicity. Still, it is important to choose your seafood wisely. There are many benefits to choosing sustainably harvested, wild seafood, both to you and to the planet.

Wild vs. farm-raised fish

Wild fish have higher levels of omega-3 fatty acids. Omega-3 fatty acids help to decrease inflammation throughout the body. Wild fish are higher in protein than farmed fish. Farmed fish has higher levels of omega-6 fatty acids, which promotes inflammation.

Farmed fish such as salmon consume food that contains cancer-causing artificial coloring to make their flesh pink. Farmed fish contain high levels of flame-retardant chemicals, pesticides, and antibiotics. Flame-retardant chemicals can interrupt the function of your hormones. The antibiotics farmed fish are fed contaminate water, leading to more antibiotic-resistant strains of bacteria threatening other sea life in the area.

Mercury contamination in fish is a problem worldwide. Mercury is toxic to every tissue in your body. It can interrupt the function of your nervous system, kidneys, lungs, and reproductive organs. Limiting exposure as much as possible is important. One way to limit the impact of mercury on your bodies is to consume ocean-caught fish rich in selenium[x]. Selenium is an antioxidant that helps decrease mercury's possible damage.

♦ Food Tool: Levels of Mercury in Seafood

Low Levels
- Anchovy
- Butterfish
- Catfish
- Clam
- Crab (domestic)

- Crawfish/crayfish
- Croaker (Atlantic)
- Flounder*
- Haddock (Atlantic)*
- Hake
- Herring
- Mackerel (North Atlantic, Chub)
- Mullet
- Oyster
- Perch (ocean)
- Plaice
- Pollock
- Salmon (wild, canned and fresh)**
- Sardine
- Scallop*
- Shad (American)
- Shrimp*
- Sole (Pacific)
- Squid (Calamari)
- Tilapia
- Trout (freshwater)
- Whitefish
- Whiting

Medium Levels
- Bass (striped, black)
- Carp
- Cod (Alaskan)*
- Croaker (White Pacific)
- Halibut (Pacific, Atlantic*)

- Jacksmelt
- Lobster
- Mahi mahi†
- Monkfish*
- Perch (freshwater)
- Sablefish
- Skate*
- Snapper*
- Tuna (canned chunk light, skipjack*†)
- Weakfish (Sea Trout)

High Levels
- Bluefish
- Grouper*
- Mackerel (Spanish, Gulf)
- Sea bass (Chilean)*
- Tuna (Yellowfin*†, canned Albacore†)

Highest Levels
- Mackerel (king)
- Marlin*†
- Orange Roughy*
- Shark*
- Swordfish*
- Tilefish*
- Tuna (Ahi*, Bigeye †)

* Overfished or caught using environmentally destructive methods

** May Contain PCBs (Polychlorinated Biphenyls)

Information from nrdc.org 2015

† Selenium-rich[XI] (Not from NRDC)

Grains, Seeds, Nuts and Legumes

All seed products must be properly prepared or they "steal" your nutrients. Seed products, grains, seeds, nuts, and legumes, have an outer layer filled with phytates and lectins, or, as I call them, vitamin chaperones. This sheath of anti-nutrients holds the vitamins and minerals inside the seed. They guard these nutrients and keep them safe until the seed sprouts.

The sprouting process liberates the nutrients so the seed can grow. If humans consume these seed products raw, or merely grind and bake them, we don't get all of the wonderful nutrients they have to offer. They pass right through us because the vitamin/chaperone combination is too large to be absorbed by our digestive systems. These anti-nutrients also inhibit our digestive enzymes and grab other free nutrients.

The highest levels of anti-nutrients are found in grains, legumes, nuts, and seeds, but there is hope. A little effort increases the availability of your nutrients. Soaking, fermenting, and sprouting are all ways to help decrease the amount of anti-nutrients in your food. Cooking grains and legumes in homemade bone stock is another great way to decrease the anti-nutrients and increase the nutritional density of your dishes.

Recipe: Soaking Grains

To soak grains, fill a quart-sized glass jar half full of the grain of your choice. Add 1 to 2 tablespoons of whey, apple cider vinegar, lemon juice, buttermilk, kefir, or yogurt to help raise the acidity level. Fill the remainder of the jar with filtered water and let it sit at room temperature for 12 to 48 hours. You can use the soak water to cook your grains, or strain and rinse the grains to remove any slight acidic taste that may remain. Soaked grains can also be dehydrated and then ground into flour if desired. Dehydrate grains until totally dry in a dehydrator or in the oven at the lowest temperature setting.

Recipe: Sprouting Grains

To sprout grains, soak grain in ample filtered water for 12 to 24 hours in a glass jar at room temperature. Drain off water and leave grain in the jar. Cover jar opening with a tight mesh or muslin cloth and place upside down at a 45-degree angle. Rinse grains three times a day with fresh water and return to the slanted position to allow excess water to drain off. Continue the daily rinsing until you see little sprouts coming out of the grain, which typically takes between two and four days. If any mold appears, compost your grains and start again.

Store sprouted grains in the refrigerator for a few days or dehydrate and store in the refrigerator for a couple of weeks. You can also grind dehydrated sprouted grain into flour and use for baking.

Recipe: Fermenting Grains

To ferment grains, fill a quart-sized glass jar half full of the grain of your choice. Add 1 to 2 tablespoons of whey, apple cider vinegar, lemon juice, buttermilk, kefir, or yogurt to help raise the acidity level. Fill the remainder of the jar with filtered water and let it sit at room temperature for 24 to 72 hours. Traditional sourdough bread is risen through this natural fermentation rather than with yeast.

Recipe: Soaking Beans

To soak beans, fill a large glass jar one-third full of beans of your choice. Add 1 to 2 tablespoons of whey, apple cider vinegar, lemon juice, buttermilk, kefir, or yogurt to help raise the acidity level. Fill the remainder of the jar with filtered water and let sit at room temperature for between 24 and 48 hours. Rinse beans well until all bubbles are gone. Cook according to your desired recipe. Skim off any foam that rises to the top while cooking.

Recipe: Soaking Seeds and Nuts

To soak seeds and nuts, fill a quart-sized glass jar half full with seeds and nuts of your choice. Add 1 to 2 teaspoons of sea salt and fill with filtered water. The water should taste salty, like the sea. Let sit at room temperature for between 12 and 24 hours. Drain off water and dehydrate nuts until crisp in a dehydrator or in the oven at the lowest temperature setting. The nuts are now ready to be used in recipes or eaten as is. Store in the refrigerator in a glass jar.

Grains and legumes to avoid

Some grains and legumes, such as processed and extruded grains, are best avoided. Processed grain products include boxed, cold cereals, cereal bars, breads and crackers. Extrusion transforms grains into different shapes, such as stars, "o's", flakes, puffs, and shreds. This process alters the proteins in the grain making them toxic to our nervous systems and kidneys.[xii] Soy is best consumed only when properly fermented and organic, as in soy sauce, miso, natto, and tempeh. Processed legumes include bean crackers and canned beans.

Fermented Foods

When I ask people what comes to mind when I mention fermented foods, beer and wine are inevitably the first ones mentioned. Yes, beer and wine are fermented, but they only make up a small portion of fermented food choices. There are other delicious options such as kefir, cheese, sauerkraut, yogurt, kimchi, and kombucha.

To be healthy, we need bacteria. These good bacteria are called probiotics—meaning pro-life. Good bacteria balance supports healthy immune, digestive, and neurologic function. Your probiotics are your body's bouncers (they keep the bad guys out) and they help break down your food, making nutrients more available for absorption. Bacteria on your skin help regulate pH, acting as a barrier to harmful pathogens. Without your bacterial friends, your susceptibility to disease increases drastically.

Probiotics must be replaced on a regular basis, and the best way to do so is through your food. Make sure you look for unpasteurized sources of these foods as pasteurization kills beneficial bacteria and the results are not nearly as nutritious. Seek to have a little fermented food with each meal.

♠ Food Tool: Food Sources of Probiotics
- Buttermilk
- Crème fraiche
- Cultured butter (made from cultured cream)
- Cultured sour cream
- Kefir (both milk and water varieties)
- Kombucha
- Miso
- Pickles (traditional, in salt-water brine rather than vinegar brine)
- Raw cheese
- Sauerkraut/kimchi/fermented vegetables of any kind
- Soy sauce (organic)
- Yogurt

Apple Cider Vinegar
Apple cider vinegar is an acidic solution produced by the fermentation of apples. Organic apple cider vinegar contains pectin and a perfect balance of 19 minerals, including potassium, phosphorus, chlorine, sodium, magnesium, calcium, sulphur, iron, fluorine, and silicon.

Recipe: Apple Cider Vinegar Digestive Primer
I like to use apple cider vinegar as a digestive primer. When taken before meals, it helps to

increase the production of digestive juices, allowing better breakdown and absorption of your food, especially the proteins. Taken before meals it can also decrease acid reflux.

Take ½ to 2 teaspoons in 4 to 6 ounces of water, 10 minutes before each meal. Sip slowly. It takes about three months of regular use before each meal to retrain your digestion with this approach. If you are irregular with your intake, it will take longer to balance, but you will still find benefit.

Sweeteners

All sweeteners, even the good ones, should be consumed occasionally at most, and in small quantities. Frequent or excessive sugar intake impacts your body's ability to heal and function properly. Most sweeteners are refined, which obliterates antioxidants and minerals, rendering them void of nutritional benefit. Even the amount of naturally occurring sugar in orange juice is enough to suppress the immune system for up to six hours.

Artificial sweeteners such as aspartame, Splenda, Equal, and NutraSweet are worse than sugar. Research links the use of artificial sweeteners to obesity, attention deficit disorder, attention deficit hyperactivity disorder, and cancer.[xiii, xiv] Avoid these as much as possible.

Some sweeteners are seemingly ubiquitous in our society, especially corn syrup and its derivatives. Corn syrup, even before it is processed to become high-fructose corn syrup, has high levels of fructose, the form of sugar most consumed in the US. Fructose is hard on your liver and difficult to process large amounts.[xv]

Another sweetener, touted as a healthy alternative to high-fructose corn syrup, is agave. Unfortunately agave, at 84 per cent fructose[xvi], has even more fructose than high-fructose corn syrup, which has 60 per cent[xvii]. Fructose in these concentrated forms increases insulin resistance, which can lead to rising triglyceride levels, increased risk of liver damage, high cholesterol levels, and increased risk of Type II Diabetes.[xviii] Agave, as well as white cane sugar and beet sugar, are highly processed and best avoided.

Sweeteners that maintain their whole food status are available. These include honey, maple syrup, date sugar, palm sugar, molasses, brown rice syrup, sucanat, and rapadura. Antioxidants and minerals are still intact in these options. Choose these when a sweetener is needed, remembering that moderation is still the key.

♠ Food Tool: Sweeteners to Enjoy, Limit, Avoid

Sweeteners to enjoy
- Coconut sugar
- Date sugar
- Honey
- Maple syrup or sugar
- Stevia

Sweeteners to limit
- Brown rice syrup
- Fruit juice concentrates
- Molasses
- Sugar alcohols—xylitol, sorbitol
- Rapadura
- Sucanat

Sweeteners to avoid
- Agave
- Aspartame
- Corn syrup or sugar
- Fructose
- Refined cane sugar– white, brown

5

Sleep:

Rejuvenate and Rebuild

Sleep is the best meditation.

~Dalai Lama

Quality sleep is necessary for deep healing to begin. People often tell me they get by just fine on four to six hours of sleep. They may be doing okay for the time being, but they are creating a severe sleep debt. Sleep, especially deep REM sleep, is when your brain makes major repairs. Large portions of the brain need to shut down to do its maintenance. If you don't allow the time to repair, you run into big problems later. Most adults are chronically sleep deprived, meaning they get 1 to 2 hours less sleep than they should each night. The effects are often not immediately obvious but compound over time.

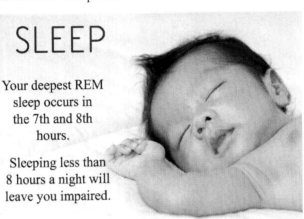

SLEEP

Your deepest REM sleep occurs in the 7th and 8th hours.

Sleeping less than 8 hours a night will leave you impaired.

Here are some questions to ask to determine your quality of sleep:

- Are you tired upon waking?
- Do you need caffeine to get and keep going?
- Do you get up in the night? If so, how many times?
- Do you snore?
- Do you need an alarm clock to wake?
- Do you wake in a very different position than when you fell asleep?
- Do you wake throughout the night?

If you answered yes to any of these questions, your quality of sleep is compromised. Waking rested and ready to go is a sign your body and mind are repairing themselves at night. Needing time to shake off sleep or requiring a cup of coffee or tea to get going is a sign you're not sleeping as deeply as needed.

Listen to your body. If you are tired take a nap, lie down in a dark room, or meditate. Ten to 20 minutes can be a great refresher. Your sleep pattern moves in 90-minute cycles. If you wish to fall asleep during your rest, consider setting an alarm for 90 minutes so you wake at the best time in the sleep cycle to feel alert and rejuvenated.

Be aware of when you're propping up your energy with sugar and caffeine. Know these will add to your energy debt and compound the problem of sleep deprivation over time.

The ideal sleep environment is in total darkness. When you're exposed to light at night, it destroys your melatonin, the hormone that helps you fall into deep sleep and stay there. Alarm clocks, smoke alarms, computers, phones, and TVs often emit light. Computers, phones, and TVs have no place in your bedroom. If you must use your cell phone as an alarm, set it to airplane mode to decrease sleep disruptions.

Creating space for deep, restful sleep
- Sleep in total darkness. Can you wave your hand in front of your face and not see movement?
- Keep your room cool.
- Keep your room quiet. If this is challenging, you may need an air purifier or another source of white noise to prevent external noises from rousing you.
- Avoid screens for between one and two hours before bed. This includes TV, computer, phone, and tablet screens.
- Remove TV and electronics from your room.
- Create a transition routine to help wind down before getting into bed. Dim the lights in your home as night falls,

step away from work, meditate, or write in a journal. This is a perfect time for your castor oil pack.

- Create a sleep routine. Go to bed and wake at the same time daily allowing enough time for a full night's sleep.

6

Hormones:

Cyclic Balance

To every thing there is a season...

~King Solomon

Hormone Basics

Every day your body and mind are in the midst of a fine orchestration of cycles and rhythms. Your hormones are big players in maintaining each cycle's balance. Hormones help balance weight, sleep, immune function, thyroid function, fertility, stress, and emotional balance, to name a few. When you are out of balance your risk of cancer, chronic disease, diabetes, and autoimmune diseases goes up. Balanced hormones allow everything to run more smoothly and regularly.

Hormone balance is off long before acute symptoms become noticeable. Your body has an amazing ability to compensate.

Here are some of the many chronic symptoms that may mean your hormones need extra support:

- Anxiety
- Brain fog
- Depression
- Digestive distress
- Excess fat storage
- Fatigue
- Fertility issues
- Frequent infections
- Hair loss or excess hair
- Headaches
- Hot flashes
- Hypertension
- Irregular menses
- Irregular moods
- Joint pain
- Low libido
- Premenstrual syndrome

- Poor concentration
- Sleep disorders
- Swelling

Hormone disruptors

Balance is a fine line to walk. Your body has multiple checks and balances to keep everything running but when other factors interrupt or block hormone creation, function, and breakdown, things can change rapidly.

Here are some of the many things that can push hormones out of balance. These factors are all dose-dependant, which means the more you are exposed, the more detrimental their effects:

- Fabric softeners
- Fire retardants in furniture, bedding, baby clothing
- Fragrances in body sprays, perfumes, fabric softeners, scented shampoos and soaps
- Heavy metals such as cadmium, mercury and lead
- Sedentary lifestyle
- Paints
- Pesticides
- Pharmaceutical antibiotics
- Phthalates in body sprays, perfumes, fabric softeners, scented shampoos and soaps
- Plastics
- Nutrient-poor diet
- Processed foods
- Prolonged intense exercise
- Soy
- Stress
- Steroids
- Styrofoam

Reducing Exposure to Toxins

While it is impossible to eliminate your exposure to hormone obstacles completely, you can greatly decrease their influence. We talked about decreasing pesticide exposure on foods with the Dirty Dozen Plus and the Clean Fifteen. It is also wise to take a look at what you put on your body as well as in it.

What is in your shampoo, toothpaste, lotion, perfume, laundry soap, dishwasher soap, and makeup? It is most likely harboring toxic ingredients. The Environmental Working Group (EWG) reviews the toxicity of cosmetics, hair, and skin care products. Skin Deep[xix] is a useful database where you can find healthier products.

Should you feel adventurous, you can easily make your own skin care products. This is a fun project to do with friends, and everyone takes home samples for spa days or daily skincare.

Quality, non-toxic skin care products can sometimes be expensive but are easily made at home. There is only one rule for healthy skin—put on your skin only what you would eat.

Cleaning your skin

Avoid using soap on your face. It removes natural oils and throws off your skin's balance. Try making your own cleansers with food-grade ingredients.

Recipe: Honey Cleanser

Raw honey is a nourishing cleanser, rich in enzymes that soothe and soften skin. Rub ½ teaspoon of honey and a drop of coconut oil or butter onto your fingertips and massage your face. Let set for 10 minutes and gently remove with a warm wet cloth.

Recipe: Oil Cleanser

Choose oils that are appropriate for your skin type.

- All skin types: Camellia, castor, coconut, kukui nut, jojoba, sunflower seed

- Normal skin: Almond, apricot kernel, camellia, coconut, jojoba, kukui nut, olive oil

- Dry skin: Almond, argan, avocado, coconut, castor, jojoba, olive, sea buckthorn berry

- Oily skin: Camellia, hazelnut, jojoba, kukui nut

Use an oil blend of your choice. Liberally apply the blend to your skin. Using slow, firm, circular motions, gently work the oil into your skin with focus on problem areas. This is a good time to practice your breathing exercises.

Soak a washcloth in hot water, as hot as you can stand. Wring out the cloth and place it on your face until it cools. Gently wipe away the oil and rinse the washcloth with hot water. Apply the hot cloth to your face, once again letting it cool. Gently wipe the remaining oil. If needed, you can rub a little oil between your palms and press it into your skin for extra hydration. Do this once or twice a week.

Recipe: Makeup Remover

Coconut oil and castor oil do a great job removing makeup and dirt. Massage the oil into your skin and gently wipe off with a soft cloth.

Polishing your skin

Exfoliate two or three times a week. Doing it too much can irritate the skin.

Recipe: Salt and Olive Oil Skin Polish

Place a ¼ teaspoon salt and 1 teaspoon olive oil in your palm. Slowly and gently massage it into your face. Avoid your eyes. Blot off with a warm cloth.

Recipe: Apple Cider Vinegar Skin Polish

Saturate a small cloth or cotton ball with apple cider vinegar and rub in circular motions around your face. Avoid your eyes. Wait two or three minutes, then blot off with a warm, wet cloth. Rinse your face with cool water.

Nourishing your skin

Oils are a great way to feed your skin. Find a mix that works for you. Everyone is different. Choose cold pressed and organic oils whenever possible.

Recipe: Facial Oil

Choose oils that are appropriate for your skin type. (See Recipe: Oil Cleanser.) In a one-ounce dropper bottle, mix a blend of your choice of oils, or use a single oil. Place one to three drops in your palm and rub together to disperse. Gently press your palms onto your face as needed.

My personal blend is about half olive oil, one quarter castor oil, and one quarter jojoba. My skin can be dry, since I live in a desert. I increase castor oil slightly in the winter.

Recipe: Lotion Bar

- 3 ounces beeswax

- 3 ounces cocoa butter

- 3 ounces oil blend (try olive, castor, coconut, jojoba, sweet almond)

- 10-15 drops essential oil (optional)

In a double boiler over low heat, melt beeswax. When melted, add cocoa butter. When the butter melts, add oil and stir until completely incorporated. Remove from heat and stir until slightly cooled, then adding essential oils.

Pour into container or molds and cool. A paper cup works well for a disposable container. Peel off just enough of the paper to use the bar while leaving a paper handhold on the opposite side. Avoid freezing as it may crack the bars. Store in a cool place. Rub all over your body-face, hands, feet, hair (as a conditioner), and lips.

Recipe: Deodorant

- 3 tablespoons shea butter

- 2 tablespoons cocoa butter

- 3 tablespoons baking soda

- 2 tablespoons arrowroot

- 5 drops essential oil (optional)

Melt butters over very low heat until almost liquid. Remove from heat and allow the last little solid butter to melt. Mix in all other ingredients. Cool the mixture so it is the consistency of porridge. Scoop into an empty, clean deodorant container and place in the fridge to firm up.

Use once to twice daily. It may take time to adjust to a new deodorant especially if you normally use antiperspirant, which this is not. I find it most effective if applied right out of the shower after drying off. This blend works well for me after trying five other versions with minimal to no success.

Balancing with Seeds

Seeds are a delicious and easy way to nourish your hormones and prevent imbalances. They are supportive for men, women, and children. If you have children in or approaching puberty, seeds can help their hormones find balance. By eating different seeds at different times of the month, you can feed your body the essential fatty acids needed to make the different hormones in your cycle.

Grind your seeds no more than a few days in advance and store extra in a glass jar in the refrigerator. Pre-ground or roasted seeds are not a good option because the oils become oxidized within a few days, rendering the fat damaging instead of nourishing. Soaking or sprouting your seeds in advance will increase their available nutrients. (For more on soaking and sprouting, see Chapter 4.)

Rotating seeds for women

Historically, women cycled with the moon. Menstruation began with the new moon and ovulation occurred on the full moon.

Seeds can help women re-establish a menstrual cycle that mimics the lunar rhythm. Then, when your cycle has stabilized, you can shift to rotating seeds according to your cycle. If your cycles are irregular, or very long or short, rotate your seeds with the lunar cycle. If you are no longer cycling due to menopause or hysterectomy, rotate your seeds with the lunar cycles.

There are apps for smartphones that send reminders of lunar phase changes and are great reminders to change your seeds. Remember, day one of your menstrual cycle is the first day of flow, not spotting. If you have a regular cycle between 25 to 29 days, rotate your seeds with your cycle. If your cycle is irregular, shorter than 25 days, or longer than 29 days rotate your seeds with the lunar cycle. If you are no longer menstruating due to menopause (natural or surgically induced), rotate with the lunar cycle. If menstruation has not yet started, rotate with the lunar cycle to ease the hormonal transition.

Recipe: From day one of your menses to day 14, or new moon to full moon

Once daily, add two tablespoons of fresh, ground, organic flax, chia or pumpkin seeds to cereals, shakes, stir-fries, rice, or anything else you are eating.

From day 15 to menses, or full moon to new moon

Once daily, add two tablespoons of fresh, ground, organic sesame or sunflower seeds to cereals, shakes, stir-fries, rice, or anything else you are eating.

Rotating seeds for men

Men benefit from rotating in the opposite cycle.

Recipe: From new moon to full moon

Once daily, add two tablespoons of fresh, ground, organic sesame or sunflower seeds to cereals, shakes, stir-fries, rice, or anything else you are eating.

From full moon to new moon

Once daily, add two tablespoons of fresh, ground, organic flax, chia, or pumpkin seeds to cereals, shakes, stir-fries, rice, or anything else you are eating.

7

Emotions:

Root Cultivation

Holding on to anger is like grasping a hot coal with the intent of throwing it at someone else; you are the one who gets burned.

~Buddha

Emotional health is a big part of overall health. Feelings can affect your physical life in the long term, and avoiding dealing with them can result in harmful effects on all the systems of the body.

Quiet time is not just for children. Breath work and silence are simple ways to get to know yourself better. The more you can cultivate this internal awareness, the easier it is to act from your true self rather than functioning in a reactive mode. Building little pockets of silence into your day makes it easier to practice your internal quiet as well. Even if it is not possible to surround yourself with silence, you can practice quieting your mind.

Emotions can sometimes feel intense and confusing. If you look at the outer manifestation of emotions, you miss about half the available information. When you evaluate a situation only by what is seen and heard externally, you inevitably make assumptions that might not be true.

There is a saying, when you "assume" you make an "ass" out of "u" and "me". Crude but true. Assumptions are the fodder for miscommunication and drama. When you become aware of your assumptions, it is easier to see clearly. When you are not clouded by your own misdirection, communicating your truth is easier and gives you a better chance of being heard.

If you are unsure how to listen to your body, start small. Focus on your hands. Do they feel warm or cold? What sensations are you aware of if you clench and release your hands? Do you feel the pressure as they close? Do you feel the small rush of warm blood as they release? Practice focusing intently on the sensations you feel to help you build internal awareness.

I have learned from personal experience. In the past, when I tried to control my emotions they would inevitably flare and backfire on me. Both my clinical practice and personal life taught me that what I resist persists.

I am not saying you should allow your emotions to control you, but rather, do not ignore your feelings. If you experience intense emotions, remove yourself from the situation and take time to assess what this emotional surge is telling you.

Tools for Emotional Health

Emotions and self-talk can sometimes seem overwhelming and deafening. When your self-talk yells at you, it can be hard to hear your true voice. In this chapter, I have collected a few simple techniques for cutting through the noise and connecting with your true self.

Nothing is ever lost when you learn something new about yourself. The more you understand where your emotions are coming from, the easier it is to step out of old patterns to find a better way to express and listen to yourself. These skills will take time to cultivate and are worth every effort.

❋ Exercise: Building Emotional Intelligence

When you feel an emotion come up, this exercise will help you investigate it.

Begin this practice in a safe quiet place. Choose a moderate or mild annoyance you currently have and feel unable to release, even though you would like to do so. It may be something you said or did, or someone else said or did. After you practice with smaller issues, move toward your deeper obstacles.

1. Identify: When you feel or imagine this emotion, where do you feel it? Where is it in your body? Try to be as clear as possible. Your breath work will help with this process. This helps you to keep the emotion in perspective and decreases the likelihood of becoming overwhelmed or lost in your emotions. Take a few deep breaths and bring awareness into your body. Bring the troubling situation into your mind. Allow yourself to feel it and explore. Start at your head and slowly work your way down as you feel this emotion. You might relive the event in your

mind to help clarify the location of the emotions associated with it in your body. Where do you find the most intense physical feelings? How much space does it fill?

2. Investigate: What does this emotion feel like? Now you have located where you feel it, draw your attention to that body part or system. Focus and put your hands over that area. You may feel constriction, numbness, pain, or shortness of breath. Lean into this feeling. Explore it without judgment. This will let your body know you are ready to let go and stop fighting or ignoring this issue.

3. Accept: Acceptance does not mean the insult or action that lead to these emotions was okay, right, or acceptable in anyway. It means you accept that this feeling exists. The emotion is valid and here to teach you something. Place your hands over the area where you feel this particular emotion, speak to that part. Say, "I acknowledge this feeling of (place your own emotion here)." Take a deep breath in and out. Then say, "I accept the existence of (insert emotion here) and am grateful for its lessons." Repeat as needed. Change the wording if desired, but keep the intent of sincere, humble exploration and surrender.

When you begin to explore your emotions and become more open to letting go, it is common for fear to arise. Fear is a good example of an emotion that instinctually makes you want to run and hide. Fear runs deep and can propel you without your conscious knowledge if you are not mindful. If you can embrace fear with compassion and love, it changes the way you interact at a core level.

This interaction goes well beyond us as individuals and impacts everyone we contact. After you become aware of your fear, it helps to reframe your perception of that fear. Viewing your fear as a frightened child can help. Imagine your fear is your frightened inner child. How would you react if a small, scared child came to you begging for comfort? Would you tell him or her to stop being scared and go away? Did it help when others said this to you? Would you gather him or her in your arms? Imagine wrapping your fearful inner child in love.

Love without judgment or expectation of return is powerful medicine. The next time you are aware of your fear, try the Building Emotional Intelligence exercise. If you meet all your emotions with compassion, you will grow.

Guided meditations

The idea of sitting quietly can be scary. You might find your mind wandering off to worry or make lists. But having something to focus on can make meditation seem more approachable, and it can also help cultivate your mental clarity. This is where guided meditations come in.

The Forgiveness Meditation, which I outline below, changed my life. It helped me let go of long-held grudges against others and myself. I first realized its efficacy in my early 20s, when I was experiencing major conflict at work with a fellow supervisor. She and I clashed from the start, which made work miserable for everyone. I tried to find my ground through meditation. After a particularly lousy day at work, I decided to meditate to cope with my anxiety about having to return the next day.

I don't know what made me do it, but at the end I gave one handful of light to this woman and one to myself. It was a mental peace offering so I didn't have to keep carrying this burden. The next day at work, our interactions were completely different. We both were mellow, cordial, and actually listened to the other. Later, we became friends and I was able to see she is a deep and beautiful person.

I also used this technique to help me let go of anger and resentment against someone who hurt me badly. Forgiveness, after all, is not for the person who has done wrong. It is for the one who forgives. The density of anger seemed to grow the longer I carried it. Continuing to carry the grudge only allowed this person to keep hurting me. I was finally ready and able to forgive.

❋ Exercise: Forgiveness Meditation

ಬಿ Find a quiet space if possible.

ಬಿ Find a comfortable position either seated or lying.

ಬಿ Place your hands on your abdomen.

ಬಿ Close your eyes and focus on your breathing.

ಬಿ Draw the air in through your nose.

ಬಿ As you inhale, your abdomen expands.

ಬಿ Exhale through your mouth like you are blowing through a straw and pull your abdomen back toward your spine.

ಬಿ Continue this for ten deep, slow, steady breaths.

ಬಿ Bring your awareness to the top of your head.

ಬಿ Scan your body from your head to your toes, being aware of any tension without judgment.

ಬಿ Draw your attention to the center of your chest, your heart.

ಬಿ Imagine a warm, nourishing light beginning to slowly grow outward from the center of your heart.

ಬಿ The healing light beckons you and you follow, drawing all your awareness to your heart.

ಬಿ Feel the warm, nourishing light wrapping and holding you, supporting and nourishing.

ಬಿ Invite the healing light into your body.

ಬಿ Allow it to fill every cell in your body, nourishing and healing.

ಬಿ As the light fills you, it displaces any old habits or thoughts that no longer serve you.

ಬ Feel the light expand and glow beyond the borders of your body.

ಬ Breathe deeply as you absorb the healing light.

ಬ Stay here as long as you need.

ಬ When every cell is full with love and healing light, extend your hands and gather two large handfuls of light.

ಬ Feel all your cells bathed in light.

ಬ Bring your thoughts to a person or situation where you feel you have been wronged or wronged someone.

ಬ Imagine them in front of you.

ಬ Offer one of your handfuls of light to their heart.

ಬ Offer the other handful to your heart.

ಬ Breathe deeply.

ಬ Gather another two handfuls of light from the endless light emanating from your heart, still filling every cell.

ಬ Repeat this offering with as many people or situations you desire.

ಬ With each offering the light within grows, as does your sense of lightness and grace.

ಬ Take a few slow, steady, deep breaths.

ಬ Notice your hands are full of light.

ಬ Take one handful and place it into your heart, feeling the light heal and soothe.

ಬ Take the other handful of light and offer it to the world.

ಬ Take just a few more slow, steady, cleansing breaths.

ಬ As you feel ready, allow the movement of one of your inhales to extend out to your fingers and toes.

ಬ Each breath brings you back.

⁕ When you are ready, allow your eyes to slowly open.

⁕ Come back into the room and back into your day.

⁕ Scan your body, being aware of any changes that occurred.

⁕ Thank yourself for allowing this time to be.

❇ Basic Deep Abdominal Exercise: Breath of Fire

Working with the breath is one way to master emotional balance. The Breath of Fire exercise, also called *agni prasana* in the yoga tradition, is designed to move everything. So be ready for change.

Breath of Fire hyper-oxygenates your body. Oxygen pushes out carbon dioxide, the waste product of all cells, and helps to shift toward balance and relaxation. This will help break loose emotional blockages and set the stage to release baggage that no longer serves you.

This is an advanced technique, so be sure to master the basic breath exercises described in Chapter 3 before moving to this exercise.

Do this technique one to 10 times a day. Slowly increase the speed of your breaths over time.

⁕ Find a comfortable seated position.

⁕ Take a slow steady breath in and out.

⁕ Close your eyes and take another slow deep breath.

⁕ Allow the breath to be driven through your abdominal movements.

⁕ Push and pull your abdominal muscles out with the inhale, in toward your spine with the exhale.

⁕ Pull your breath forcefully in and out through your nose.

⁕ Do 30 rapid and rhythmic breaths.

⁕ Sit quietly for 30 seconds.

8

Grounding:

Building a Foundation

*Let the gentle bush dig its root deep and
spread upward to split the boulder.*

~Carl Sandburg

We are electrical beings and benefit from grounding, both electrically and emotionally.

How do you know you are not grounded? You can have obvious physical symptoms such as dizziness, headaches, chronic upper respiratory tract infections, or vertigo. Mental symptoms may manifest as a feeling of being stuck in your thoughts and emotions. These are all signs that grounding exercises will help.

Electrically speaking, your heart sets your rhythm. Science has long known that emotions can affect the heart's rate and rhythm. The heart sends more information to the brain than the brain sends to the heart, and each emotion is associated with different heart rhythms. These electrical signals change when you focus on gratitude and compassion by becoming longer and smoother.[xx] There is emotional information in these signals that impacts your sense of wellbeing and that of those around us. Have you ever walked into a room after someone was arguing? What did the atmosphere feel like? What changed in your body at that moment? There is a saying that you could "cut the tension with a knife" in these situations. That tension comes from the "charge" in the room.

One of the simplest ways to help you ground is to sit in the grass with your shoes off. Place your hands and feet directly on the earth. As an electrical being, you carry a charge, and so does the earth. The earth will literally ground you and bring your charge closer to an ideal neutral.

Here is an exercise you can do anywhere—inside or outside—to help you ground and connect. Sitting on the earth for this exercise makes it even better.

✳ Exercise: Get Grounded

- ཀྵ Find a quiet space if possible.
- ཀྵ Find a comfortable position either seated or lying.
- ཀྵ Place your hands on your abdomen.
- ཀྵ Close your eyes and focus on your breathing.
- ཀྵ Draw the air in through your nose.

- ❧ As you inhale your abdomen expands.

- ❧ Exhale through your mouth like you are blowing through a straw and pull your abdomen back toward your spine.

- ❧ Continue this for ten deep slow steady breaths.

- ❧ Draw your awareness to just below your belly button.

- ❧ Maintain your awareness in your lower abdomen as you feel roots beginning to extend down from the soles of your feet.

- ❧ Feel your roots delving down through the dirt and rocks.

- ❧ Down through the bedrock.

- ❧ Down into the deep stream of cool nourishing water.

- ❧ Feel the stable presence of earth balancing the steady flow of water.

- ❧ Draw up nourishment and energy from the water and earth.

- ❧ All the way up your roots, through your toes, up your legs, trunk, arms, and head.

- ❧ The flow displaces all that no longer serves you and washes it out to be recycled by the earth.

- ❧ Continue to breathe deeply and slowly.

- ❧ Stay here for as long as you wish.

- ❧ Feel the nourishment displacing unnecessary baggage.

- ❧ Take a slow deep breath in and out.

- ❧ Slowly begin to find movement in your toes and fingers.

- ❧ Take another deep breath in and out.

- ❧ When you are ready, slowly open your eyes.

- ❧ Come back into the room and back into your day.

- ❧ Thank yourself for allowing this time to ground.

9

Movement:
One Step at a Time

Just play. Have fun. Enjoy the game.

~Michael Jordan

Regular movement is very important. This does not have to be super-intense or take hours every day. A little goes a long way. Even 30 minutes of gentle walking is shown to decrease stress hormones and increase metabolic function.

MOVEMENT

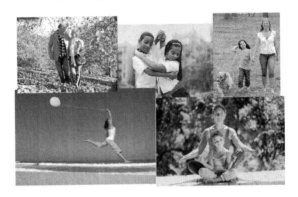

Start small by walking around the block, doing a sun salutation, parking a few spots further away from work, or taking the stairs. Increasing your activity is not about buying a gym membership or expensive equipment, but if these help inspire you, by all means, use them. Find a walking buddy or someone with whom to take dance lessons. Have fun with it and better yet, get outside. Aim for at least 30 minutes a day.

Excessively intense or prolonged exercise can take a toll on your system over time. Moderation and balance is key. Consider Tai Chi, Yoga, walking, hiking, swimming, biking, or Qi Gong to help balance your central nervous system and get your body moving.

Rest:

The Art of Inaction

Sit in reverie and watch the changing color of the waves that break upon the idle seashore of the mind.

~Henry Wadsworth Longfellow

Sometimes action, no matter the intent, causes harm. We all need physical, mental, emotional, and spiritual breaks. All things need rest to rejuvenate. We see this in the growth of spring and summer to the slowing and hibernation of fall and winter. This is part of the seasonal cycle.

The art of pause in these middle moments holds the juice of life. The collective consciousness of our society holds the belief that to do nothing is unproductive. This shows in the phrase "idle hands are the devil's workshop." It implies if you are not *doing* something, trouble ensues.

I used to feel guilty for taking time for self-care and even more so when it involved me just being. After graduating from naturopathic medical school and passing my board exams, I crashed. Without having a monster to-do list sitting on me, I didn't know what to do with myself. I thought I should be doing something, but my mind and body required deep rest. Even the thought of small chores brought me to tears. So I hibernated, sleeping 12 to 18 hours a day for two months. This is where I learned the art and necessity of therapeutic nothingness.

After I paid back my sleep debt and rebuilt some of my energy stores, I was able to function again. Without the downtime void of intellectual and physical stimulation, I would have driven myself deeper into adrenal fatigue. During rest is when you heal, rebuild, and grow mentally, physically, emotionally, and spiritually.

Allow yourself time for therapeutic nothingness. In fact, schedule it into your life. I like to have at least one day a week where I don't have anything scheduled. This helps me feel like I'm not constantly running from one thing to another.

Conclusion

Stumbling or falling do not equal failure.
They are lessons teaching us how to walk, run,
jump, and ultimately, dance.

~Dr. Allegra

You are your best teacher. Listen to what your body and mind are telling you. Lean into it and explore without judgment. Know you are love. You are connected to everything around you. Everything implying separation and isolation is delusion.

The changes we discussed in this book don't come overnight. This journey is made up of many steps. Each step and breath is an opportunity to reset and begin again. Just because you made a less-than-ideal choice in the past doesn't mean you must continue in a direction that no longer serves you. Guilt over past choices will get you nowhere and is not worth your time and energy.

Now that you have more knowledge about how to better care for yourself you can make better choices. Making better choices with the information you have takes practice. Practice implies there is a strong likelihood you will need to repeat each step over and over before you get it right a majority of the time.

After you have made self-care a daily habit, it becomes much easier, but it is still a conscious practice. In reality, you will fall down, and you will fail, but none of that matters. All that matters is that you get back up and try again. That is what defines who you are. Give yourself kudos for each step you take and celebrate each little step.

You can do this.

Take one step and one breath at a time. You will thrive!

Index of Exercises

Index of Food Tools

Index of Recipes

Recommended Reading

A New Earth: Awakening to Your Life's Purpose. Eckhart Tolle

Deep Nutrition: Why Your Genes Need Traditional Food. Catherine Shanahan and Luke Shanahan

Eat Fat Lose Fat: The Healthy Alternative to Trans Fats. Mary Enig and Sally Fallon

Nourishing Traditions: The Cookbook that Challenges Politically Correct Nutrition and the Diet Dictocrats . Mary Enig and Sally Fallon

Nutrition and Physical Degeneration. Weston A. Price

Wild Fermentation: The Flavor, Nutrition, and Craft of Live Culture Foods. Sandor Ellix Katz

Ramiel Nagel "Living with Phytic Acid" Wise Traditions. (Spring 2010)

Resources
Crunchybetty.com: Natural skin and hair care recipes

Ewg.org: Skin Deep database and annual Dirty Dozen Plus

Greenpasture.org: Fermented Cod Liver Oil

Mountainroseherbs.com: Herbs, oils, salts, butters

Naturaeclinic.com: Guided meditations and self-care resources

Realmilk.com/real-milk-finder: Clean raw milk international options

Westonaprice.org: Weston A. Price Foundation

Endnotes

[i] McGarey MD, William. The Oil That Heals: A Physician's Successes With Castor Oil Treatments. A.R.E. Press, 1993.

[ii] Sears CL (October 2005). "A dynamic partnership: celebrating our gut flora." *Anaerobe* 11 (5): 247–51.

[iii] Guarner F, Malagelada JR (February 2003). "Gut flora in health and disease." *Lancet* 361 (9356): 512–9

[iv] *Population Health Metrics* 2010, **8**:29 doi:10.1186/1478-7954-8-29

[v] http://www.cdc.gov/ncbddd/autism/data.html

[vi] Jeffery M. Smith. Genetic roulette: the documented health risks of genetically engineered foods. Yes! Books, 2007.

[vii] http://responsibletechnology.org/health-risks

[viii] http://www.ewg.org/foodnews/list.php

[ix] Pathophysiology. 2015 Mar;22(1):39-48. doi: 10.1016/j.pathophys.2014.12.001. Epub 2014 Dec 13.

[x] *Neurotoxicology.* 2008 Sep;29(5):802-11. doi: 10.1016/j. neuro.2008.07.007. Epub 2008 Aug 9.

[xi] http://www.wpcouncil.org

[xii] *Cereal Chemistry,* American Association of Cereal Chemists, Mar/Apr 1998 V 75 (2) pp. 217-221

[xiii] Trends Endocrinol Metab. 2013 Sep;24(9):431-41. doi: 10.1016/j.tem.2013.05.005. Epub 2013 Jul 10.

[xiv] Eur J Clin Nutr. 2008 Apr;62(4):451-62. Epub 2007 Aug 8.

[xv] Am J Clin Nutr. 2014 Oct;100(4):1133-8. doi: 10.3945/ ajcn.114.086074. Epub 2014 Aug 6.

[xvi] J Agric Food Chem. 2012 Sep 5;60(35):8745-54. doi: 10.1021/jf3027342. Epub 2012 Aug 21.

[xvii] Nutrition. 2014 Jul-Aug;30(7-8):928-35. doi: 10.1016/j. nut.2014.04.003. Epub 2014 Apr 18.

[xviii] J Clin Endocrinol Metab. 2014 Jun;99(6):2164-72. doi: 10.1210/jc.2013-3856. Epub 2014 Mar 6.

[xix] Skin Deep Database: http://www.ewg.org/skindeep/

[xx] http://www.heartmath.com/personal-use/emwave-science-behind.html

About the Author

Dr. Allegra Hart is a physician, author, and teacher with a successful naturopathic clinic. Her goal is to help you rebuild your health from the inside out. She specializes in taking you on a journey through self-care and nourishment to optimum health, empowering you with more energy, better digestion and moods, and increased flexibility in meeting stressful situations. Learn more at naturaeclinic.com.

38722819R00055

Made in the USA
San Bernardino, CA
11 September 2016